Mohamed Amine Baba
Ahmed Kharbach

Nursing students and healthcare-associated infections

Mohamed Amine Baba
Ahmed Kharbach

Nursing students and healthcare-associated infections

Healthcare-associated infections

ScienciaScripts

Imprint

Any brand names and product names mentioned in this book are subject to trademark, brand or patent protection and are trademarks or registered trademarks of their respective holders. The use of brand names, product names, common names, trade names, product descriptions etc. even without a particular marking in this work is in no way to be construed to mean that such names may be regarded as unrestricted in respect of trademark and brand protection legislation and could thus be used by anyone.

Cover image: www.ingimage.com

This book is a translation from the original published under ISBN 978-620-3-45681-3.

Publisher:
Sciencia Scripts
is a trademark of
Dodo Books Indian Ocean Ltd. and OmniScriptum S.R.L publishing group

120 High Road, East Finchley, London, N2 9ED, United Kingdom
Str. Armeneasca 28/1, office 1, Chisinau MD-2012, Republic of Moldova, Europe
Printed at: see last page
ISBN: 978-620-6-09876-8

Knowledge, Attitudes and Practices of Nursing students regarding nosocomial infections

Mr Mohamed Amine BABA

Kharbach Ahmed

Dedication

From the depths of my heart, I dedicate this work to all those who are dear to me,

To my parents, my wife, my son

To my brothers and sisters.

To my dear friends

Summary

The level of knowledge of nosocomial infections is an essential component in the enhancement of measures to combat nosocomial infections and in the development of effective preventive and curative strategies. The aim of this study is to describe the state of knowledge, attitudes and practices of nursing students with regard to healthcare-associated infections.

This was a cross-sectional study, using a self-administered questionnaire, which took place between February and June 2019. One hundred and fifty-nine students (n=159) were surveyed. The mean score for general knowledge was 3.42 ± 1.50. The mean score for knowledge of attitudes and practices was 11.50 ± 3.42. The average total score was 14.92 ± 5.007. The total score was higher for students who had received training in nosocomial infections (P<0 .05). The Multi-skilled Nurse option recorded the best knowledge scores compared with the other options in the pathway. The definition of nosocomial infection and the mode of transmission by hand were ignored by more than half the students. Bacteria were the most frequently cited microbial agent in relation to nosocomial infections. Almost all the students were unaware of the regulatory aspect. The management of excreta and the prevention of HAIs were the most neglected standard precautions.

In the light of the results obtained and the literature, a number of recommendations and suggestions have been made to improve student nurses' knowledge, attitudes and practices with regard to healthcare-associated infections.

Table of contents

I.   Introduction

Infections that occur in hospitals are known as hospital-associated infections. These infections are also called "nosocomial infections" and sometimes "hospital-acquired infections". As outpatient care is increasingly provided to ambulatory patients, the term "healthcare-associated infections" is also used. (organisation, 2002)

Hospital-acquired infections represent a real public health problem, due to their frequency, severity, and also their socio-economic cost (World Health Organization, 2017). Moreover, hospital-acquired infection is the result of the provision of unsafe care (Allegranzi et al., 2011). In the same perspective, the World Health Organisation (WHO) revealed that on average 8.7% of hospitalised patients had acquired a nosocomial infection (Organization, 2005) and that developing countries are up to 20 times more likely to contract a nosocomial infection than developed countries.

According to the WHO, the prevalence rate of nosocomial infection in Morocco is 17.8 (WHO, 2009) . Although infection is most common in patients on admission, healthcare professionals also act as potential vectors of pathogens. Hospitals are a favourable transmission route for the spread of nosocomial infections, partly due to poor infection control practices among healthcare workers and patient overcrowding in most clinical settings(Samuel et al., 2010) .

These infections are generally caused by a number of factors, including environmental factors such as the cleanliness of instruments, floors and walls and antimicrobial resistance, as well as factors related to the knowledge and attitudes of healthcare staff with regard to infection prevention. (Ward, 2011)

As a result, and in order to deal with these factors, which are linked to staff knowledge, the World Health Organisation (WHO) recommends programmes to combat nosocomial infections, which must be very comprehensive and cover both surveillance and prevention activities and staff training. In this respect, prevention and monitoring alone do not guarantee their reduction without good training of healthcare workers. In this respect, a study carried out in western Algeria revealed that the lack of compliance with standard precautions aimed at preventing the transmission of infectious agents via blood and body fluids was mainly due to a lack of knowledge (Benali Beghdadli et al., 2008) .

One component of care workers are nursing students who are exposed to the hospital environment during their clinical placement and are obliged to provide care to patients, regardless of their disease status (AL-Rawajfah & Tubaishat, 2015) thus the limited clinical experience of novice nurses with regard to routine precautions, their lack of knowledge of the use of personal protective equipment, and inadequate training in clinical procedures are contributing factors to the increased risk of nosocomial infections (AL-Rawajfah & Tubaishat, 2015).

A study conducted in Saudi Arabia (Amin et al., 2013) assessed medical students' knowledge and behaviour regarding the standard precautionary principle and infection control. Most students (80.0%) felt that there was an urgent need for training in infection control and 61.4% felt that their current medical curriculum did not provide sufficient information.

Other cross-sectional surveys of nursing students in Africa have also shown that the majority of this population have poor knowledge, attitudes and practices regarding nosocomial infection control measures.(Ojulong, Mitonga, & Iipinge, 2013) and that a structured educational programme was needed (Thakker, Jadhav, & care, 2015)

A study by J Ojulong, KH Mitonga and SN Iipinge concluded that there is a need to improve or revise the curriculum to ensure that health science students' knowledge of infection prevention and control is communicated promptly prior to their introduction to wards (Ojulong et al., 2013). A study by Ajediran I Bello et al concluded that the students sampled demonstrated moderate knowledge of hospital-acquired infections, acquired mainly through theoretical classroom training. These findings highlight the need for greater emphasis on education about this important source of infection in the clinical training curriculum (Bello et al., 2011)

The role of student nurses in the patient safety process and in ensuring their own protection during training courses is still poorly understood in Morocco. The aim of this study is therefore to explore the knowledge of nursing students about the risk of infection and the rules of precaution, hand hygiene and barriers to ensure patient safety and the self-protection of nursing students.

With this in mind, we proposed to launch a survey to establish the level of knowledge of nursing students about nosocomial infections and to deduce the actions to be implemented to reinforce their basic training.

Consequently, the objective of this study is to explore the state of knowledge, attitudes and practices relating to nosocomial infections among nursing students at the Institut Supérieur des Professions Infirmière et Techniques de Santé d'Agadir. In particular, (i) to explore the general knowledge of students in the care stream about nosocomial infections and (ii) to explore the knowledge of students in the care stream in terms of attitudes and practices for the prevention of nosocomial infections.

II. Literature review

2.1 General information on nosocomial infections

2.1.1 Definition of nosocomial infection

Nosocomial infections are defined as infections that appear during or following hospitalisation and are not present, either during incubation or on admission to hospital. When the infectious state on admission is not known, a delay of at least 48 hours after admission (or a delay greater than the incubation period when this is known) is commonly accepted to distinguish a nosocomial acquisition infection from a community-acquired infection(Murthy et al., 2016).For surgical site infections, infections occurring within 30 days of the operation or, if an implant, prosthesis or prosthetic device is used, within one year of the operation, are generally considered to be associated with the care provided. (Beaucaire, 1997).

Nosocomial infections can involve all types of infectious agents, but they are most frequently bacterial, and more occasionally viral, fungal or parasitic. (Pozzetto, 2004). Nosocomial infections are infections contracted in a healthcare establishment. This definition, taken from the "100 recommendations for the surveillance and prevention of nosocomial infections" published in 1999, was updated in November 2006 by the French Technical Committee on Nosocomial Infections and Healthcare-Related Infections. Nosocomial infections are now included in healthcare-associated infections (HAIs). An infection is considered to be a HCAI if it occurs during or after the provision of care (diagnostic, therapeutic, palliative, preventive or educational) to a patient, and if it was neither present nor incubating at the start of the care. Nosocomial infections affect patients, whether ill or not, but also healthcare professionals and visitors (CTINILS, 2006).

There are several types of hospital-acquired infection with different modes of transmission:

- Infections of "endogenous" origin: the patient infects himself with his own micro-organisms, through an invasive procedure and/or because of a particular fragility.

- Infections of "exogenous" origin: the micro-organisms originate from other patients (cross transmission between patients or by the hands or equipment of staff), staff or contamination of the hospital environment (water, air, equipment, food, etc.). (Durocher, 2005).

2.1.2 Factors favouring nosocomial infection:

Whatever the mode of transmission, the occurrence of a nosocomial infection is favoured by the patient's medical situation, which depends on :

- Age and pathology: the elderly, immunocompromised people, newborns (especially premature babies), polytrauma victims and burn victims are particularly susceptible.

- Certain treatments (antibiotics that unbalance patients' bacterial flora and select resistant bacteria; immunosuppressive treatments);

- Carrying out invasive procedures necessary for patient treatment: urinary catheterisation, catheter placement, artificial ventilation or surgery, etc.

Medical advances have made it possible to care for increasingly fragile patients who often have a number of risk factors. This means that these risk factors must be taken into account when interpreting the rates of nosocomial infections measured in epidemiological surveys.

Preventing hospital-acquired infections is a complex task, because most of them depend on a number of factors. While it is difficult to control all the factors linked to the medical situation of patients given the current state of our knowledge, the quality of care and the safety of the hospital environment must be the subject of reinforced vigilance and preventive action. (Durocher, 2005).

2.1.3   Chain of transmission of infection

The infection transmission chain is made up of six links: the infectious agent, the reservoir, the exit route, the mode of transmission, the entry route and the receptive host. Transmission occurs when all six elements of the transmission chain are present. Transmission can be prevented by breaking any of the links in this chain (PHAC, 2018) :

<u>The infectious agent</u>

It is a transmissible micro-organism. It may be a bacterium, a virus, a fungus, a parasite or a prion. It belongs either to the endogenous flora (the individual's own microorganisms) or to the exogenous flora (the user's external source).

The reservoir or source

A user, healthcare worker or visitor who may have an active infection, be asymptomatic, be incubating an infectious disease, or be transiently or chronically colonised by a pathogenic micro-organism.

Microorganisms

They can be found on the skin, in blood, biological fluids, excretions and secretions, etc. The inanimate environment or care equipment shared from one user to another can also be a reservoir and a source of nosocomial infections.

The way out

This is the route by which the infectious agent leaves the reservoir, although not all reservoirs have an obvious exit point. When the reservoir is associated with a host, it may be the anatomical site through which the microorganism leaves the reservoir. For example, this could be the respiratory tract, which expels contaminated secretions when sneezing or coughing. It could also be a break in the skin with bleeding or a wound with exudate. When the reservoir is associated with the environment, the exit route may be more difficult to identify.

Mode of transmission

This is the means by which the infectious agent reaches the receptive host, from the source. A distinction is made between transmission by contact (physical contact or via an inanimate object), by droplets (large respirable particles travelling over a distance of up to two metres), by air (small particles travelling over long distances), by a common vehicle (contaminated source) or by a vector. The mode of transmission varies according to the type of microorganism. In addition, some infectious agents can be transmitted by more than one route. The portal of entry is the route by which an infectious agent enters a host. Entry points include mucous membranes (e.g. respiratory tract), the genital tract, the gastrointestinal tract, the urinary tract, skin lesions (e.g. wounds) and invasive devices such as intravenous catheters.

The receptive host

A person who is receptive to the infectious agent (microorganism) either, for example, because their immune system is weakened or they lack the antibodies needed to fight the infection, or because they have the appropriate cellular receptors to host the agent.

<u>Preventing the transmission of infections</u>

To prevent the transmission of infections, all you have to do is break one or other of these links. A good way of doing this is to apply effective infection prevention and control measures, in a hierarchical fashion, by first trying to control the source of the infection. Vaccination is another example of a preventive measure.

2.2. Standard precautions

Standard precautions (SP) are the basis for preventing the cross-transmission of micro-organisms. They have proven their effectiveness and represent the first barrier measures to be respected. They must be known and applied for all care, in all places, for all patients, whatever their infection status, and by all healthcare professionals.

In the mid-1970s, the introduction of the concept of PS represented a major innovation in the prevention of healthcare-associated infectious risks (Beaucaire, 1997) In 2017, following the development of knowledge and practices, the French Society of Hospital Hygiene (SF2H) updated the recommendations on standard precautions so that they can be applied to all care, in all places, for all patients, whatever their infection status, and by all healthcare professionals.

The SF2H recommendations can be broken down into six areas (SF2H, 2017):

- Hand hygiene.

- Personal protective equipment.

- Respiratory hygiene **(new).**

- Prevention of accidents involving exposure to blood or any biological product of human origin.

- Excreta management **(new).**

- Environmental management.

2.2.1 Hand hygiene

During care, hand hygiene is indicated because there is a risk of transferring micro-organisms from the skin of a patient/resident or from one surface to another. Transmission via the contaminated hands of healthcare staff is the most common form of transmission in most healthcare facilities. The five WHO guidelines for hand hygiene during care:

1. before contact with the patient,

2. before an aseptic procedure,

3. after a risk of exposure to a biological product of human origin,

4. after contact with the patient,

5. after contact with the patient's environment

Hand hygiene is carried out using two techniques:

1. Disinfection by friction with a hydroalcoholic product is the benchmark technique because it is: more effective and faster at inactivating micro-organisms, better tolerated by the skin than washing with soap and water, and the benchmark for all hand hygiene indications in the absence of visible soiling. The recommended time for disinfection by friction is 30 seconds. (Bloc, Dupuis, Massardier, Gaucherand, & Doret, 2010)

2. Within the scope of standard precautions, the only situations in which simple hand washing with water and mild soap remains recommended are: in the event of accidental contact with a biological product of human origin, and in the event of visibly soiled hands (glove powder or other visible soiling).The recommended time for hand washing is a minimum of 15 seconds(SF2H, 2017).

2.2.2 Personal protective equipment

Personal protective equipment (PPE) refers to the following barrier measures

- Wearing gloves

- Face protection (mask/glasses)

- Protection of the outfit.

Used alone or in combination, PPE protects healthcare professionals from the risk of exposure to micro-organisms during contact with mucous membranes, injured skin, and in the event of contact or risk of contact with a biological product.(SF2H, 2017)

<u>Wearing care gloves</u>

o Wear gloves only: if there is a risk of exposure to blood or any other biological product of human origin, contact with mucous membranes or damaged skin or during care if there are skin lesions on the hands of the carer.

o Gloves should be put on just before the treatment and removed and discarded immediately afterwards. Gloves should be changed between two patients and between two treatments (**1 glove = 1 patient = 1 treatment).** (Chaib et al., 2016)

<u>Face protection :</u>

Wear a medical mask and safety goggles or a face shield if there is a risk of exposure by splashing or aerosolisation to a biological product of human origin.

<u>Protection of the outfit :</u>

✓ Shape

The shape should be simple, comfortable and ergonomic, with short sleeves. The length is adapted to the wearer. The fastenings should not have the usual buttonholes or cuffs, to avoid collecting "contaminating dust". Fastening is by press studs.(B Beghdadli, Kandouci, Ghomari, Dagorne, & Fanello, 2007)

✓ Pace of change

Work clothes must be changed daily and whenever they become soiled. When taking meals, it is replaced by street clothes in order to protect it from soiling and limit the risks of transmission of micro-organisms which it carries. In the event of major exposure to biological products of human origin: a single-use, long-sleeved, waterproof gown must be worn, and the protection put on just before the procedure, and removed immediately at the end of a care sequence and between two patients.

2.2.3 Respiratory hygiene :

Any person (patient, resident, visitor, healthcare professional, outside worker, carer, etc.) presenting respiratory symptoms such as coughing or expectoration should wear a mask. It is important to carry out hand hygiene after contact with respiratory secretions or contaminated objects. Do not touch mucous membranes (eyes, nose, mouth) with contaminated hands.

2.2.4 Prevention of accidents involving exposure to blood or any biological product of human origin :

- For care using a perforating object: Care gloves must be worn and the medical safety devices provided must be used after use. Any perforating object must not be recapped, bent, broken or even removed from the hand.

If the object is single-use, it must be disposed of immediately after use in a suitable container for perforating objects, located as close as possible to the treatment. In the case of reusable objects, the equipment must be handled with care and cleaned and disinfected quickly. For treatment involving a risk of projection/aerosolisation, wear appropriate personal protective equipment (face protection, protective clothing, gloves if the skin is damaged).

2.2.5 Excreta management:

It is essential to wear appropriate personal protective equipment (care gloves, protective clothing) and to observe hand hygiene when handling excreta (urine, faeces, vomit). Manual procedures for emptying and cleaning containers should be avoided, and rinsing should be avoided (no showers or hand showers) because of the risk of aerosolisation.

2.2.6 Environmental management

Any material (medical devices, linen, waste, etc.) visibly soiled or potentially contaminated by blood or any other biological product of human origin must be handled using appropriate personal protective equipment.

<u>Reusable medical equipment or devices :</u>

 Before use, check that the equipment has undergone an appropriate maintenance procedure at the required level (non-critical, semi-critical, critical). After use, clean and/or disinfect the equipment using an appropriate procedure.

<u>Soiled linen and waste :</u>

It is essential to dispose of the waste as soon as possible after the treatment, in a closed bag and using the appropriate channel. Next, clean and/or disinfect the patient's immediate environment (bedside table, adaptor, bed, etc.), frequently used surfaces (door handles, sanitary facilities, etc.) and premises (floors, surfaces) according to appropriate procedures and frequency.

2.3 Students' knowledge, attitudes and practices regarding nosocomial infections

2.3.1 General knowledge of nosocomial infections

Several studies have assessed students' general knowledge of nosocomial infections. In particular, this assessment concerned: the definition of nosocomial infection, the factors involved, the reservoir, the receptive host, the modes of transmission and the germs responsible for this infection.

Some studies have shown that students have little knowledge of the definition of nosocomial infection (Hien et al., 2013; Kra, Aoussi, Ehui, Ouattara, & Bissagnéné, 2009; Trop, 2008) Most of them are unaware of the minimum 48-hour period required to distinguish between community-acquired and nosocomial infections. The same results were obtained in a study of two groups of doctors and nurses, with only 6.4% to 16.5% of those interviewed able to answer correctly. (DE YOPOUGON, 2007). On the other hand, a study carried out in Africa showed that the reservoir, the receptive host and the modes of transmission were less well known (Kra et al., 2009) .

Furthermore, the importance of the role of the hand in the occurrence of nosocomial infections has been highlighted in the literature. It is estimated that between 20% and 40% of nosocomial infections are due to the manual transmission of an infectious agent (Loczenski, 2005) However, only 6% of student nurses cited hand-carried transmission(Kra et al., 2009)On the other hand, another study of healthcare professionals showed that only 39.3% of those surveyed stated that the patient contracted a nosocomial infection by being hand-carried (Hien et al., 2013) . For the microbial agent responsible for nosocomial infection. It has been shown that HIV, HBV and HCV, viruses that can be transmitted during HAI, were rarely cited by students, but bacterial agents were the most frequently mentioned. (Kra et al., 2009) .

In a study carried out in Dakar, which included the regulatory aspect of nosocomial infection among the knowledge that students and healthcare workers should have, only 1/3 of healthcare workers who had correctly answered the question of the nosocomial infection control committee (CLIN) (Trop, 2008) . Another study showed that 71.6% of the staff interviewed were unaware of the existence of the hygiene and nosocomial infection control committee (DE YOPOUGON, 2007).

2.3.2   Knowledge of attitudes and practices to prevent nosocomial infections

To assess knowledge relating to the attitudes and practices of healthcare workers, the majority of studies have been based on standard precautions drawn up either by the WHO or by learned societies. Among the recommendation guides, we find that of the French Society of Hospital Hygiene (SF2H), which presents a latest update of these recommendations concerning standard precautions. (SF2H, 2017)

In fact, several studies have explored the knowledge of carers and students about standard precautions. In this respect, a study carried out among students revealed a high rate of between (60% and 90%) correct answers on the value of standard precautions among the groups surveyed (Rahiman, Chikte, & Hughes, 2018) . A survey of doctors showed that 76.2% were able to correctly define standard precautions. With regard to standard precautions, doctors and medical laboratory scientists showed a good knowledge of hand hygiene as a standard precaution in both groups surveyed, but respiratory hygiene was rarely mentioned. (Ndu & Arinze-Onyia, 2017). .

In Morocco, fifth-year medical students showed a good knowledge of the indications for hand hygiene (Razine et al., 2009) the same result obtained in another study (Ogoina et al., 2015) .

Some studies among carers have shown a low awareness of different types of hand washing, despite their recognition that wearing gloves does not exclude hand washing.(Hien et al., 2013) . A similar result was found among medical school students, where almost half of externals (46%) did not know the difference between simple washing and antiseptic washing. The same study revealed that the majority of respondents stated that the short-sleeved gown is recommended in the care environment; they also stated that they change their gown every three and a half weeks except in the case of a task, where the change is made on average after three days. (Duroy & Le Coutour, 2010)

III. Methods :

3.1 Type of study

This is a descriptive, cross-sectional study that took place between March and June 2019
.

3.2 Study environment

The study will take place at the Institut Supérieur des Professions Infirmière et Techniques de Santé in Agadir.

3.3 Target population

students in the care programme at the Institut Supérieur des Professions Infirmières et Techniques de Santé d'Agadir, and in accordance with the ISPITS founding decree (ISPITS, 2013)The nursing (SI) stream comprises five options:

IP	Multi-skilled nurse
IAR	Anaesthetic and intensive care nurse
ISFSC	Family and Community Health Nurse
ISM	Mental health nurse
ISUSI	Emergency and Intensive Care Nurse

3.4 Inclusion and exclusion criteria

They are included in this study. Students in semester four and semester six.

The number of care students registered for the spring session of the 2018 / 2019 academic year by option and semester is as follows: (Table 1)

Table 1 Distribution of students in different options by semester of training

Option	IP	IAR	ISFSC	ISM	ISUSI	Total
4ème Semester	33	22	17	22	13	**107**
6ème Semester	20	15	14	13	00	**62**
Total	53	37	31	35	13	**169**

Source: ISPITSA Student Affairs Unit.

3.5 Sampling method

In this study, the researcher opted for an exhaustive census. The aim is to improve the representativeness of the sample.

3.6 Data collection

A self-administered questionnaire was used to assess students' knowledge. This questionnaire was sent to all IS students present on the day of the survey. The questionnaire consisted of 27 questions divided into two sections: i) general knowledge of healthcare-associated infections. ii) knowledge of attitudes and practices to prevent nosocomial infections.

A repository of recommendations updated in 2017 for the surveillance and prevention of healthcare-associated infections was used to identify variables (SF2H, 2017).

Knowledge score

A Knowledge Score was used to assess general knowledge and knowledge of attitudes and practices relating to hospital-acquired infections.

We set a knowledge score as follows (Appendix 1)

A total score out of 30, including 10 points for general knowledge of nosocomial infections and 20 points for knowledge of attitudes and practices to prevent nosocomial infections.

A total score interpretation scale was presented as follows:

- A total score of 0 to 9 is considered as a level of knowledge: Low

- A total score of 10 to 19 is considered a level of knowledge: Medium

- A total score of 20 to 30 is considered a level of knowledge: Good

3.7 Statistical analysis

- The data collected was analysed using SPSS.25 software.

- The margin of error is calculated for a confidence level of 95%.

- Quantitative variables were expressed as mean ± standard deviation.

- Qualitative variables are presented in tables of numbers and frequencies

- The Chi-squared test was used to determine the correlation between the categorical variables

- The ANOVA test was used for the correlation between the quantitative variables

3.8 Ethical and regulatory considerations

Authorisation to conduct the study was obtained from the Institut Supérieur des Professions Infirmières et Techniques de Santé. Consent was obtained from the students for their participation in the study. The data were collected, entered and processed anonymously. (See survey sheet)

IV. Results:

4.1 Population characteristics:

In this survey, one hundred and fifty-nine nursing students (n=159) were questioned. This represents a participation rate of 94.08% (Table 2).

Table 2 Study participants by option

Option	IP[1]	IAR[2]	ISFCS[3]	ISM[4]	ISUSI[5]	Total
Frequency	52	35	24	35	13	**159**
Percentage (%)	32,7	22,0	15,1	22,0	8,2	**100**

Analysis of the results showed that the average age of the participants was 20.74 ± 1.04 years, with a minimum age of 18 and a maximum age of 25. Females predominated, with a sex ratio of 0.35.

According to an analysis of the course descriptions for the IS options, 76 students (47.79%) had taken a course on nosocomial infections as part of their basic training.

4.2 Knowledge score:

The majority of students, 88.7%, obtained an unsatisfactory general knowledge score (<5). In addition, half of the students had a below-average Attitudes and Practices score (<10). Overall, the total score was less than or equal to 15 for 58% of students. (Table 3)

The best general knowledge scores, attitude and practice scores, and total scores were recorded in the IP option and in the group that underwent nosocomial infection training.

A significant difference between numbers of hospital placements and knowledge scores ($P<0.05$). (Table 4)

---

[1] Multi-skilled nurse
[2] Anaesthetic and intensive care nurse
[3] Family and Community Health Nurse
[4] Mental Health Nurse
[5] Emergency and Intensive Care Nurse

Table 3 Average and median knowledge scores of students in the Nursing programme

Knowledge scores	Mean ± Σ	Median	Extremes [Lower terminal, Upper terminal].
General knowledge score ‡	3,42 ±1,503	3,00	[1 ,7]
Knowledge of attitudes and practices score £	11,50 ± 3,866	11,00	[6 ,18]
Total score ¥	14,92 ± 5,007	14,00	[7 ,24]

‡ Score for general knowledge is out of 10; £ score for knowledge of attitudes and practices is out of 20; ¥ total score is out of 30.

Table 4 Breakdown of students' knowledge scores by option, course and number of placements

	Score connaissances générale Moyenne ± Σ	P Value	Score connaissance des attitudes et pratiques Moyenne ± Σ	P value	Score Total Moyenne ± Σ	P value
Options :		0,001		<0,001		<0,001
IP	4,90 ±1,142		15,79 ±1,786		20,69 ±2,02473	
IAR	2,40 ±0,976		8,71 ±2,217		11,14 ± 2,64734	
ISFSC	2,83 ±1,274		11,83 ±3,002		14,66 ± 4,11431	
ISM	2,91 ±0,951		8,77 ±2,302		11,68 ± 2,80516	
ISUSI	2,69 ±1,109		8,54 ±1,808		11,23 ± 2,58695	
Suivi d'une formation en matière d'IN		<0,001		<0,001		<0,001
Oui	4,25 ±1,524		14,54 ±2,891		18,78 ±3,99104	
Non	2,66 ±1,003		8,71 ±2,173		11,38 ±2,68615	
Nombre de stage hospitalier		0,002		<0,001		<0,001
Inf. ou égal à 3	3,77 ±1,503		12,81 ±3,717		6,56 ±4,760	
Entre 4 et 6	3,28 ±1,454		10,57 ±3,683		13,88 ± 4,83312	
> 6	2,08 ±,760		8,46 ±2,537		10,53 ± 3,12558	

IP Multi-skilled nurse
IAR Anaesthesia and Intensive Care Nurse
FHCS Family and Community Health Nurse
ISM Mental Health Nurse
ISUSI Emergency and Intensive Care Nurse

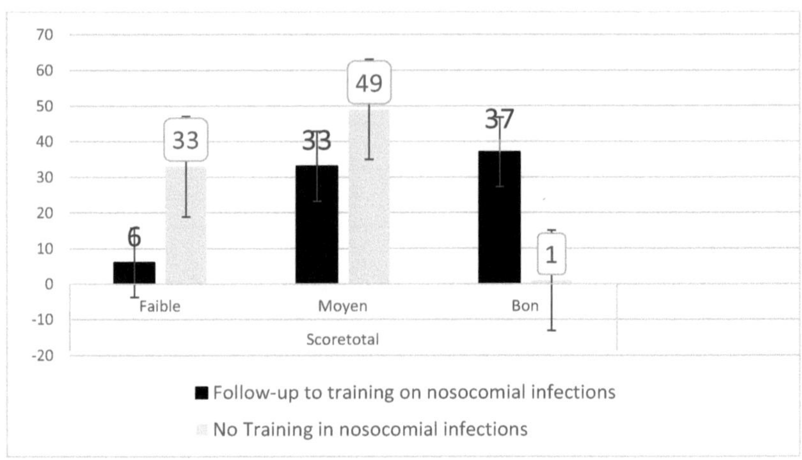

Figure 2: Total score for student knowledge according to course taken

The majority of students who had received training in nosocomial infection had a good level compared with those who had not, with a highly significant difference between the two groups (KI SQUARE value of P< 0.001) (Figure 4).

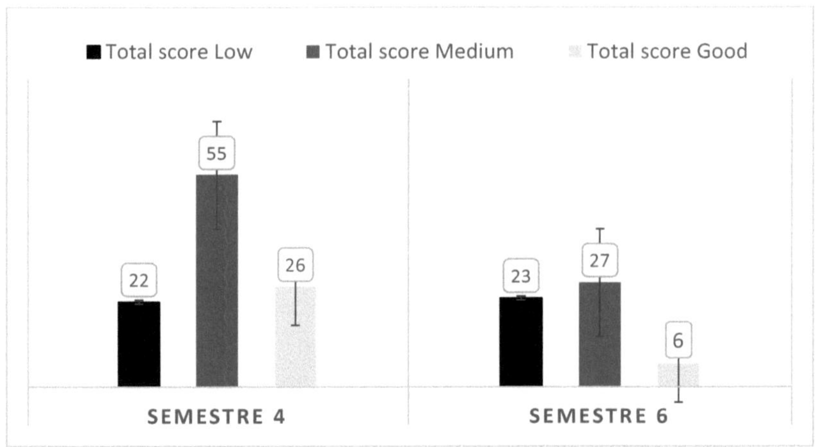

Figure 3: Distribution of total knowledge scores by semester of study

The total score of students in semester four is better than that of students in semester six (Figure 5).

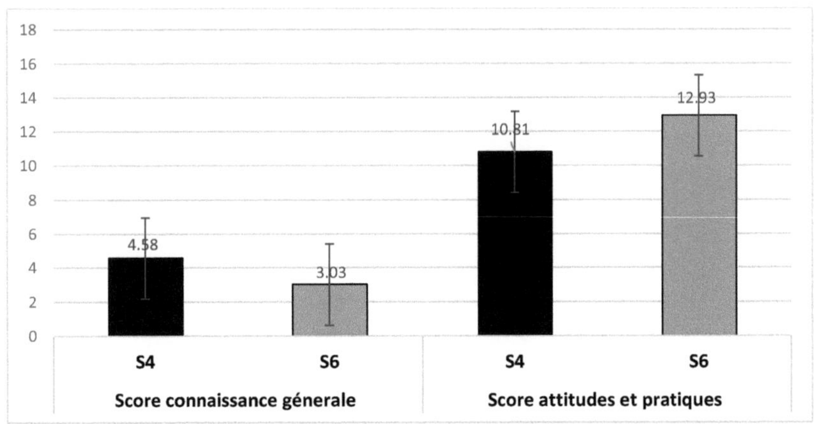

Figure 4: Average score for general knowledge and average score for knowledge of attitudes and practices, by semester of study

For the general knowledge score, students in semester four obtained a higher score than students in semester six, but for the knowledge of attitudes and practices score, students in semester six obtained the highest score (Figure 6).

4.3. General knowledge of nosocomial infections

The frequencies of responses in relation to general knowledge of nosocomial infection are shown in table 5 :

Table 5 Distribution of students' responses concerning the various elements of general knowledge relating to hospital-acquired infections

Questions	Number (Percentage)
Definition of IN	
True	66 (41,5 %)
Fake	**93** (58,5 %)
Reported risk factors :	
≤ 2 factors	74 (46,5 %)
> 2 factors	**79** (49,7 %)
No factors	6 (3,8 %)
Manual transmission method	
Yes	54 (34,0%)
No	**105** (66,0%)
IN is not transmissible	
Yes	12 (7,5 %)
No	**147** (92,5)
IN receptive host	
Full answer	75 (47,2%)
Incomplete answer	**84** (52,8 %)
IN reservoir	
Full answer	69 (43,4 %)
Incomplete answer	**89** (56,0 %)
Bacteria responsible for IN	
Yes	**148** (93,1 %
No	11 (6,9 %)
Virus responsible for IN	
Yes	77 (48,4 %)
No	**82** (51,6 %)
Parasite is responsible for IN	
Yes	**104** (65,4 %)
No	55 (34,6 %)
Mushroom is responsible for IN	
Yes	**84** (52,8 %)
No	75 (47,2 %)

More than half of the nursing students were unaware of the more precise definition of nosocomial infection, which takes into account the time required for hospitalisation (Table 5). However, the majority of correct answers were recorded among students in the multi-purpose option and the majority of incorrect answers in the mental health option (Table 6). The difference between the options is therefore considered significant. (Chi-square value of 0.001).

The transmissible nature of the nosocomial infection was well known in 92.5% of cases. (Table 5). The role of the hand in the occurrence of nosocomial infections was ignored by 66% of the students surveyed, with only the multi-skilled students having a high percentage of correct answers, whereas almost all ISUS and ISFSC students did not mention the hand-carried mode (Table 6).

As for the reservoir of this infection, 56.0% of IS students had incomplete answers (Table 6). In addition, their knowledge of the host of nosocomial infection was poor.

With regard to the microbial agents responsible for nosocomial infection, the majority of students attributed the infection to bacterial agents, whereas viruses were rarely cited in most responses. (Table 6)

Table 6 Distribution of general knowledge by training option

Questions	PI n (%)	IAR n (%)	GSSI n (%)	ISM n (%)	ISUS n (%)	P value
Definition of IN						0,000
True	**50**	**15**	**12** (13,0%)	**6** (6,5%)	**9** (9,8%)	
Fake	(54,3%)	(16,3%)	**12** (17,9%)	**29**	**4** (6,0%)	
	2	**20**		(43,3%)		0,001
Reported risk factors :	(3,0%)	(29,9%)				
			17 (23,0%)		9 (12,2%)	
≤ 2 factors			7 (8,9%)	**22**	4 (5,1%)	
> 2 factors	**16**	**10**	00,0%	(29,7%)	**0**	
No factors	(21,6%)	(13,5%)		**12**		
	35	**21**		(15,2%)		0,000
Manual transmission method	(44,3%)	(26,6%)		**1** (16,7%)		
	1	**4** (66,7%)	**2** (3,7%)		**3** (5,6%)	
Yes	(16,7%)		**22** (21,0%)		**10** (9,5%)	
No				**8** (14,8%)		0,131
		6 (11,1%)		**27**		
IN is not <u>**transmissible**</u>	**35**	**29**	**4** (33,3%)	(25,7%)	**0** (0,0%)	
Yes	(64,8%)	(27,6%)	**20** (13,6%)		**13** (8,8%)	
No	**17**					
	(16,2%)					0,469
			13 (17,3%)	**4** (33,3%)	**4** (5,3%)	
IN receptive host		**3** (25,0%)	**11** (13,1%)	**31**	**9** (10,7%)	
Full answer		**32**		(21,1%)		
Incomplete	**1** (8,3%)	(21,8%)				0,034
answer	**51**		**12** (17,4%)		**4** (5,8%)	
	(34,7%)		**12** (13,5%)	**16**	**9** (10,1%)	
IN reservoir		**14**		(21,3%)		
Full answer		(18,7%)		**19**		0,079
Incomplete	**28**	**21**	**22** (14,9%)	(22,6%)	**13** (8,8%)	
answer	(37,3%)	(25,0%)	**2** (18,2%)		**0** (0,0%)	
	24					
Bacteria responsible for IN	(28,6%)	**9** (13,0%)		**12** (17,4%)		0,000
Yes		**26**	**5** (6,5%)	**23**	**2** (2,6%)	
No	**32**	(29,2%)	**19** (23,2%)	(25,8%)	**11**(13,4%)	
	(46,4%)					0,000
Virus responsible for IN	**19**	**29**		**34**		
Yes	(21,3%)	(19,6%)	**7** (6,7%)	(23,0%)	**8** (7,7%)	
No		**6** (54,5%)	**17** (30,9%)	**1** (9,1%)	**5** (9,1%)	0,002
	50					
Parasite is responsible for IN	(33,8%)					
	2					
Yes	(19,6%)	**11**	**8** (9,5%)	**11**	**7** (8,3%)	
No		(14,3%)	**16** (21,3%)	(14,3%)	**6** (8,0%)	
		24		**24**		
Mushroom is responsible for IN		(29,3%)		(29,3%)		
Yes	**48**					
No	(62,3%)					
	4 (4,9%)					
		21		**25**		
		(20,2%)		(24,0%)		
		14		**10**		
	43	(25,5%)		(18,2%)		
	(41,3%)					
	9					
	(16,4%)					
		19		**12**		
		(22,6%)		(14,3%)		

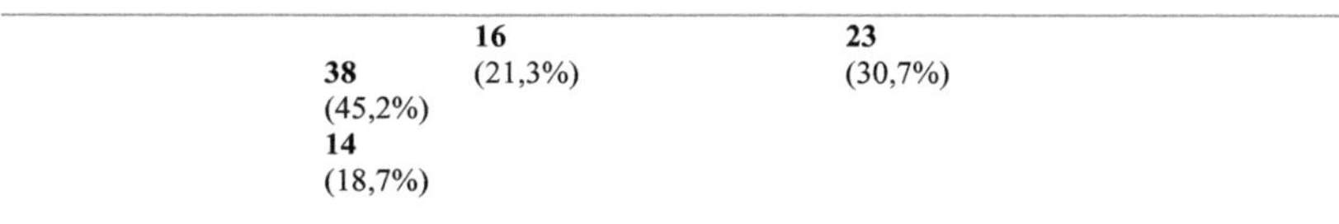

38 (45,2%)	**16** (21,3%)	**23** (30,7%)
14 (18,7%)		

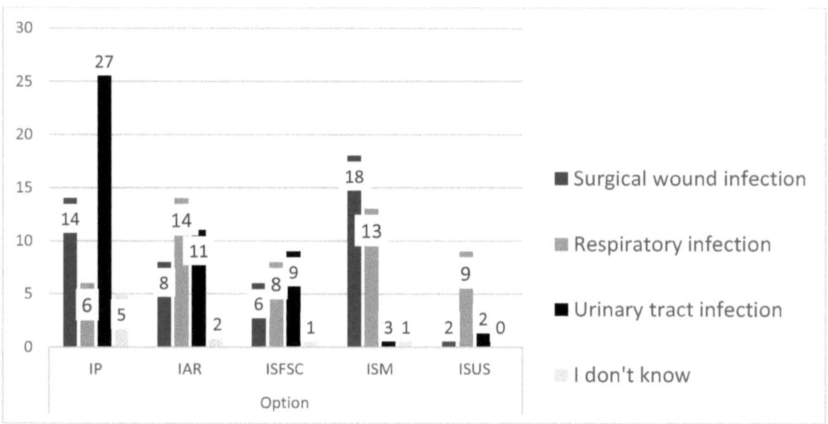

Figure 5: Distribution of knowledge of the most common nosocomial infection according to training options

The declaration of urinary tract infection as the most common nosocomial infection in our context is very marked in the responses of students in the IP (Multi-skilled nurse) option, with significant incorrect responses more specifically among students in the ISUS and ISM options.

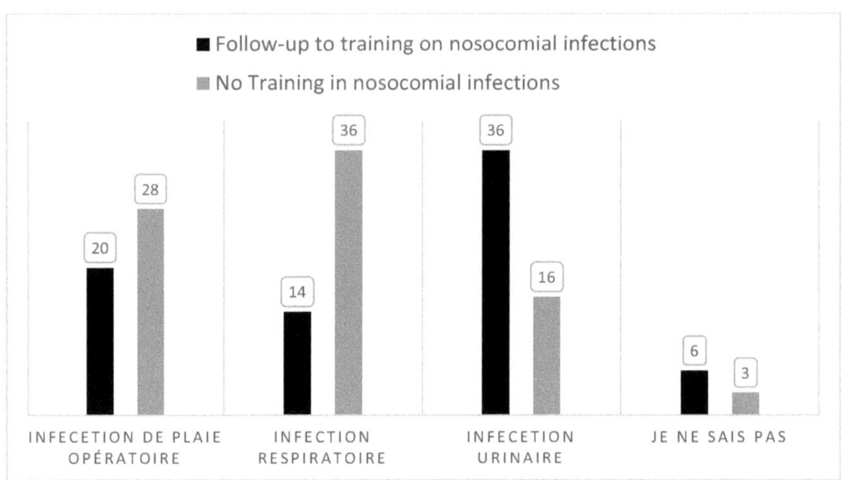

Figure 6: Distribution of knowledge of the most common nosocomial infection according to completion of nosocomial infection training .

Students who had already received training in nosocomial infection showed good knowledge of the most common nosocomial infection, compared with those who had not, with a difference between the two groups that was highly significant (Chi-square value of 0.000).

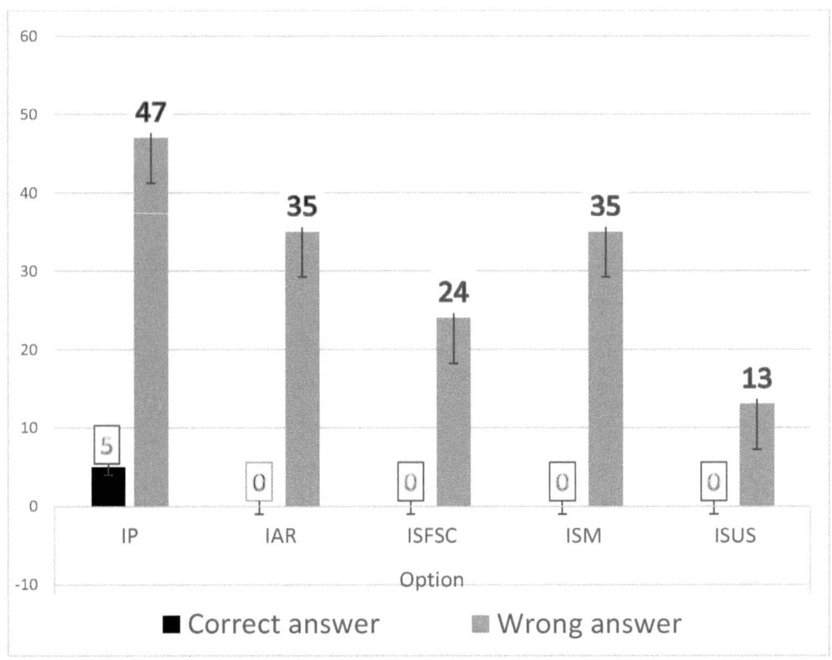

Figure 7: Students' awareness of the body responsible for preventing hospital-acquired infections, by training option

The nosocomial infection control committee (CLIN), which is considered to be the hospital body responsible for preventing nosocomial infections, was not known by the majority of students in the IS stream; in fact, the five correct answers were recorded by students in the multi-skilled nursing option.

IP Multi-skilled nurse
IAR Anaesthesia and Intensive Care Nurse
FCHS Family and Community Health Nurse
ISM Mental Health Nurse
ISUSI Emergency and Intensive Care Nurse

4.4 Knowledge of attitudes and practices to prevent nosocomial infections

Table 7 Distribution of student responses regarding knowledge, attitudes and practices in the prevention of hospital-acquired infections

Questions	Number (Percentage)
The value of standard precautions :	
True	130 (81,8 %)
False	28 (17,6 %)
Standard precautions include :	
Hand hygiene	
Yes	139 (87,4 %)
No	20 (12,6 %)
Excreta management	
Yes	36 (22,6 %)
No	123 (77,4%)
Environmental management	
Yes	99 (62,3 %)
No	60 (37,7 %)
AES prevention	
Yes	67 (42,1 %)
No	92 (57,9 %)
Indication for hand hygiene :	
True	67 (42,1 %)
Fake	92 (57,9 %)
Keep gloves on between treatments	
Yes	60 (37,7 %)
No	99 (62,3 %)
Wash hands before wearing gloves	
Yes	
No	113 (71,1%)
	46 (28,9 %)

Table 8 Distribution of knowledge of attitudes and practices by option

Questions	PI n (%)	IAR n (%)	GSSI n (%)	ISM n (%)	ISUSI n (%)	P value
The value of standard precautions :						**0,002**
True	**48**	**31**	14 (10,8%)	**25**	12 (9,2%)	
False	(36,9%)	(23,8%)	10 (35,7%)	(19,2%)	1 (3,6%)	
Standard precautions include :	**4**	**4**		**9**		
	(14,3%)	(14,3%)		(32,1%)		**0,013**
Hand hygiene						
Yes			23 (16,5%)		12 (8,6%)	
No			1 (5,0%)		1 (5,0%)	
	50	**26**		**28**		
Excreta management	(36,0%)	(18,7%)		(20,1%)		**0 ,000**
Yes	**2**	**9**	3 (8,3%)	**7**	**00** (0,0%)	
No	(10,0%)	(45,0%)	21 (17,1%)	(35,0%)	**13**	
					(10,6%)	**0,040**
Environmental management	**22**	2 (5,6%)	13 (8,2%)	**9**		
Yes	(61,1%)	**33**	11 (6,9%)	(25,0%)	9 (5,7%)	
No	**30**	(26,8%)		**26**	4 (2,5%)	
	(24,4%)			(21,1%)		0,229
			9 (13,4%)			
AES prevention		**15**	15 (16,3%)		8 (11,9%)	
Yes	**37**	(9,4%)		**25**	5 (5,4%)	
No	(23,3%)	**20**		(15,7%)		**0,000**
	15	(12,6%)	8 (11,9%)	**10**		
Indication for hand hygiene :	(9,4%)		16 (17,4%)	(6,3%)	**2** (3,0%)	
					11	
True		**10**			(12,0%)	**0,000**
Fake	**25**	(14,9%)		**15**		
	(37,3%)	**25**	10 (16,7%)	(22,4%)		
Keep gloves on between treatments	**27**	(27,2%)	14 (14,1%)	**20**		
Yes	(29,3%)			(21,7%)	9 (15,0%)	
No					4 (4,0%)	**0,007**
	35	**9** (13,4%)		**13**		
Wash hands before wearing gloves	(52,2%)	**26**	16 (14,2%)	(19,4%)		
Yes	**17**	(28,3%)	8 (17,4%)	**20**		
No	(18,5%)			(23,9%)	10 (8,8%)	
					3 (6,5%)	
	7	**10** (16,7%)		**24**		
	(11,7%)	**25**		(40,0%)		
	45	(25,3%)		**11**		
	(45,5%)			(11,1%)		
	46	**19** (16,8%)		**22**		
	(40,7%)	**16**		(19,5%)		
	6	(34,8%)		**13**		
	(13,0%)			(28,3%)		

The healthcare students surveyed had a good knowledge of the importance of applying standard precautions to protect patients and healthcare workers, with a significant difference between the options (chi-square value of 0.002).

Almost all of the IS students considered hand hygiene to be one of the standard precautions. Regarding the management of excreta, it was found that students were not very familiar with this measure, with a glaring figure among students in the ISUSI option, none of whom mentioned this measure as one of the standard precautions.

Half of the IP students were familiar with the indications for hand hygiene, compared with the other options, where knowledge was low, especially among ISUSI students.

The responses from ISM mental health students show poor knowledge of the recommended attitude for wearing gloves, with the majority stating that it is recommended to keep them on between treatments.

Washing hands before wearing gloves was well known in almost all the responses from students in all the care pathway options.

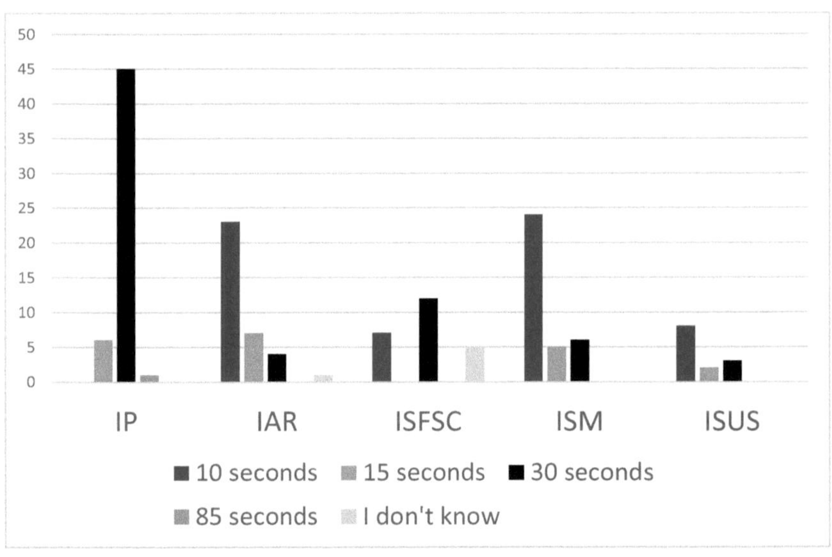

Figure 8: Students' knowledge of the recommended time for applying an alcohol-based disinfectant

Students in the multi-purpose option were well aware of the recommended time for applying hygienic hand rub (Figure 10), whereas students in the ISM and IAR options showed little awareness.

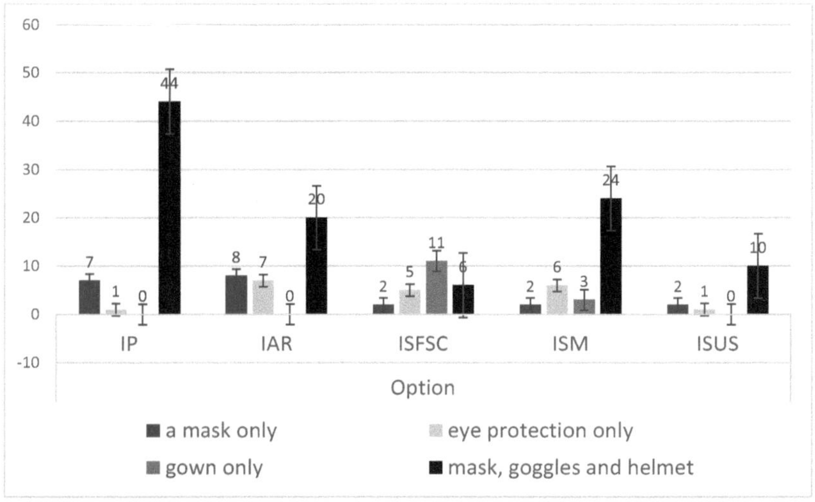

Figure 9: Knowledge of personal protective equipment in the event of risk of splashing or spraying of blood or biological fluids

Most students in the IS stream were well aware of the need to wear personal protective equipment (masks, goggles and glasses) in the event of blood or body fluids being splashed or sprayed (Figure 11), while students in the ISFSC option were less aware.

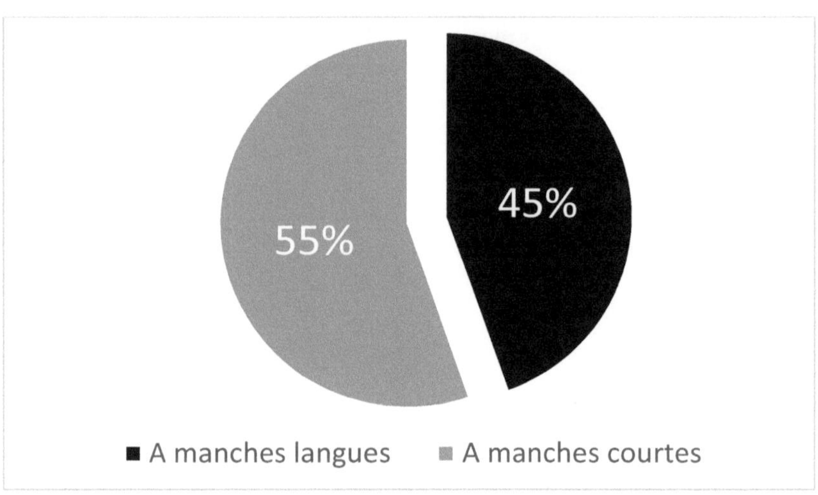

Figure 10: Shape of gown recommended for carers according to students

Less than half of IS students say that the recommended shape for nursing gowns should be long-sleeved.

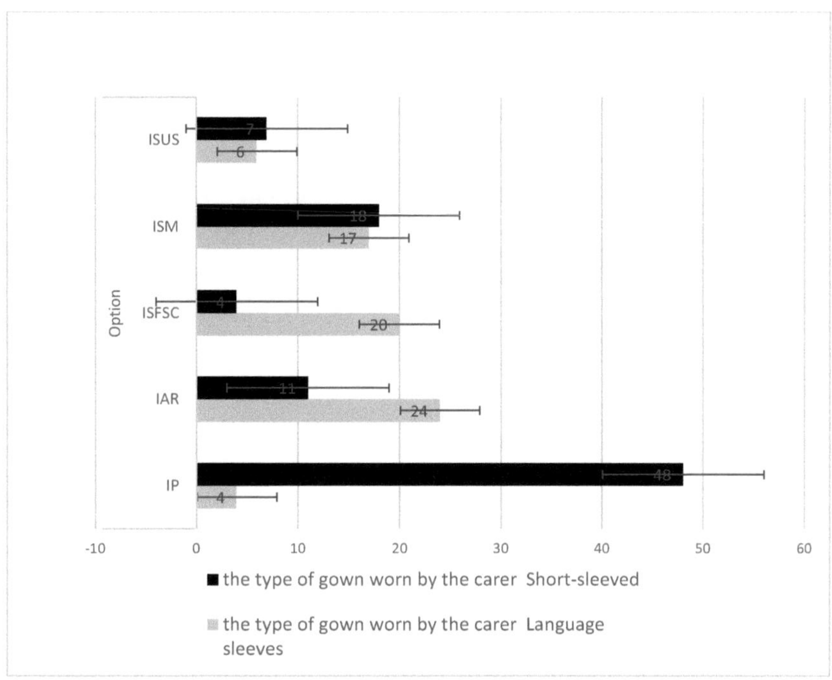

Figure 11: Knowledge of recommended gown shape for carers by training option

The majority of ISFSC and IAR students were unaware of the recommended type of gown to be worn by the carer, compared with 92.30% of IP students who said they were familiar with this attitude.

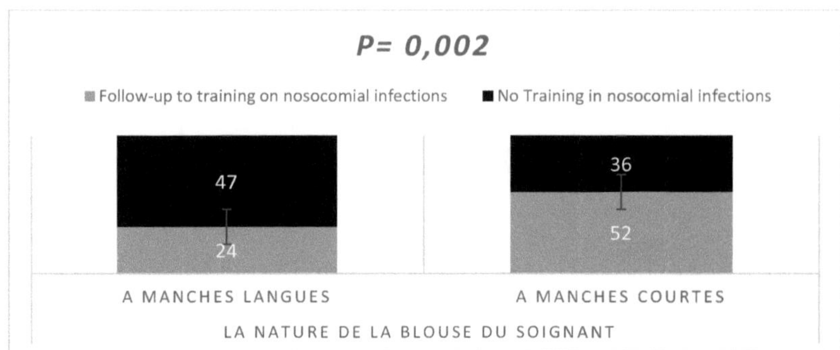

Figure 12: Knowledge of the recommended shape of the gown for carers, according to training received

However, the group that had already received training on nosocomial infection had a better understanding of the recommendation to wear a short-sleeved gown than the group that had not, with a significant difference between the two groups *(P = 0.002).*

V. Discussion

Our study is based on a "knowledge, attitudes and practices" survey on nosocomial infections. A number of findings emerged from our assessment of the state of knowledge in our student community, and our results corroborate those found in other international studies.

The main findings were in favour of a better total knowledge score for students who had already undergone basic training in nosocomial infection. The same result was obtained in recent research that showed an improvement in the knowledge of students participating in an online training module on standard precautions to prevent nosocomial infections (Hassan, 2018).

In terms of knowledge levels by semester, the overall score was higher for students in semester four than in semester six. This may be due to the fact that students in the latter group are less likely to remember course content relating to hospital-acquired infections. As for the different knowledge inherent in attitudes and practices, a better score was noted among students in the sixth semester. This could be explained by the greater number of clinical placements compared with students in the fourth semester. This is in line with a similar study which showed that among nurses, the attitudes and practices score increases proportionally with the years of practice (Hien et al., 2013).

In terms of general knowledge, 58.5% of the students gave a correct definition of nosocomial infections. The transmissible nature of HAI was well known by almost all participants (92.5%). These results are similar to those of other studies, which found a 98% correct response rate for nosocomial infections and a satisfactory level of knowledge of the definition of nosocomial infections among students. (Kra et al., 2009). On the other hand, a modest level of knowledge of the epidemiological chain was identified in our investigation. This is also corroborated by the study by Kra (2009) (Kra et al., 2009). It is therefore clear that it will be difficult for these student nurses to take preventive action if they lack knowledge of the epidemiological chain and modes of transmission.

In fact, only a third of the students recognised the hand-me-down mode of transmission. However, this percentage is much higher than that described by Kra and colleagues, who reported only 6%. (Kra et al., 2009). The importance of the role of the hand in the occurrence of nosocomial infections is emphasised in the literature, and it is estimated that 30% to 40% of nosocomial infections are due to the hand-carried transmission of an infectious agent (Loczenski, 2005).

In our study, the majority of students mentioned bacteria as the microbial agent responsible for nosocomial infection, whereas 51.6% did not mention viruses. This is in line with a similar study showing a good knowledge of student nurses, especially of bacterial agents compared with the other agents responsible for nosocomial infection (Kra et al., 2009).

Almost all the students in the care stream were unaware of the nosocomial infection control committee as the body responsible for preventing nosocomial infections in hospitals. However, another study showed that the CLIN was correctly recognised by a third of students (Trop, 2008). In our context, this finding could be explained by the fact that the regulatory aspect is not integrated into the course taught to students.

The integration of standard precautionary measures to prevent NI is of crucial importance in the routine practice of nursing professionals in order to ensure their protection and that of their patients (Liu, Curtis, & Crookes, 2014). In this respect, the majority of student responses linked the importance of standard precautions with the protection of patients and all healthcare workers. The same results were obtained elsewhere, with a high rate of between 60% and 90% of correct answers on the value of standard precautions (Rahiman et al., 2018). In Nigeria, on the other hand, a study showed that only 34.2% of patients had heard of standard/universal precautions (Ofili, Asuzu, & Okojie, 2003).

Our survey also revealed a low level of student knowledge of excreta management and respiratory hygiene, as two standard precautions, even among students who had already received training in nosocomial infection. This may be explained by the fact that the content taught is not up to date.

Student nurses who had received training were well aware of the need for hand hygiene, compared with those who had not. The same observation was made in a study of 5th year medical students (Razine et al., 2009) while in another study, the three groups surveyed showed a low level of knowledge of the indications for hand hygiene (Ogoina et al., 2015) . Knowing that wearing gloves does not exclude hand washing, the participating students showed good knowledge in this respect. As was shown in another study of novice nurses (Hien et al., 2013) .

The carer's gown should be plain, comfortable, ergonomic with short sleeves, so almost 44.7% failed to respond to the nature of the recommended gown for carers, in contrast to the study by Hien and colleagues which showed that 87.5% of student nurses mentioned the short-sleeved gown (Hien et al., 2013).

Conclusion

The results of this study revealed an unsatisfactory level of knowledge about nosocomial infections, particularly in relation to the epidemiological chain and the regulatory aspect. A much greater gap was found between students who had not received training in nosocomial infection and the trained group.

The integration of theoretical and clinical training modules is very important in order to anchor good practice and attitudes to the prevention and control of nosocomial infections in the day-to-day practice of student nurses. Similarly, continuing education programmes, through the organisation of seminars, symposia and workshops for student trainees, are also essential in order to keep abreast of the latest recommendations from learned societies.

Indeed, more effort is needed to improve or revise training curricula so that nursing students' knowledge of infection prevention and control is improved.

This investigation was limited by the evaluation of the behavioural and attitudinal aspect only at the theoretical level. As a result, further studies evaluating students' behaviours and attitudes to NI empirically via participant observation are crucial to demystifying the hidden facet of nursing trainees' current practices in the various hospital placements.

Bibliography

AL-Rawajfah, O. M., & Tubaishat, A. J. N. e. t. (2015). Nursing students' knowledge and practices of standard precautions: a Jordanian web-based survey. *35*(12), 1175-1180.

Allegranzi, B., Nejad, S. B., Combescure, C., Graafmans, W., Attar, H., Donaldson, L., & Pittet, D. J. T. L. (2011). Burden of endemic health-care-associated infection in developing countries: systematic review and meta-analysis. *377*(9761), 228-241.

Amin, T. T., Al Noaim, K. I., Saad, M. A. B., Al Malhm, T. A., Al Mulhim, A. A., & Al Awas, M. A. J. G. j. o. h. s. (2013). Standard precautions and infection control, medical students' knowledge and behavior at a Saudi university: the need for change. *5*(4), 114.

PHAC. (2018). Public Health Agency of Canada "Infection prevention and control basics: transmission chain of nosocomial infection".

Beaucaire, G. J. L. r. d. p. (1997). Nosocomial infections: Epidemiology, diagnostic criteria, prevention, principles of treatment. *47*(2), 201-209.

Beghdadli, B., Belhadj, Z., Chabane, W., Ghomari, O., Kandouci, A. B., & Fanello, S. J. S. P. (2008). Compliance with "standard precautions" by nursing staff at a university hospital in western Algeria. *20*(5), 445-453.

Beghdadli, B., Kandouci, A.-B., Ghomari, O., Dagorne, C., & Fanello, S. J. A. d. M. P. e. d. l. E. (2007). Manipulation des cytostatiques: quels risques pour le personnel infirmier du CHU de Sidi-Bel-Abbès. *68*(4), 414-419.

Bello, A. I., Asiedu, E. N., Adegoke, B. O., Quartey, J. N., Appiah-Kubi, K. O., & Owusu-Ansah, B. J. I. j. o. g. m. (2011). Nosocomial infections: knowledge and source of information among clinical health care students in Ghana. *4*, 571.

Bloc, F., Dupuis, O., Massardier, J., Gaucherand, P., & Doret, M. J. J. d. G. O. e. B. d. l. R. (2010). Are caesareans abused in extreme emergencies? , *39*(2), 133-138.

Chaib, Y., ELanssari, A., Aouane, M., Hamama, S., Oujar, N., Chakhtoura, K., ... Studies, A. (2016). The factors related to the patients hospitalized favoured nosocomial infections. *14*(2), 472.

CTINILS, I. C. T. f. d. I. N. e. d. I. L. a. S. (2006). 100 recommendations for the surveillance and prevention of nosocomial infections.

DE YOPOUGON, C. J. R. B.-A.-N. S. (2007). EVALUATION OF THE LEVEL OF KNOWLEDGE AND PRACTICAL ATTITUDES CONCERNING NOSOCOMIAL INFECTIONS AT THE UNIVERSITY HOSPITAL OF YOPOUGON, DURING 2006. 52-56.

Durocher, A. J. S. s. e. s. (2005). L'infection nosocomiale comme indicateur de (non) qualité des soins: l'exemple de la réanimation (Commentary). *23*(3), 59-68.

Duroy, E., & Le Coutour, X. J. M. e. m. i. (2010). Hospital hygiene and medical students. *40*(9), 530-536.

Hassan, Z. M. J. A. j. o. i. c. (2018). Improving knowledge and compliance with infection control Standard Precautions among undergraduate nursing students in Jordan. *46*(3), 297-302.

Hien, H., Drabo, M., Ouédraogo, L., Konfé, S., Sanou, D., Zéba, S., ... Méda, N. J. S. P. (2013). Knowledge and practices of healthcare professionals on healthcare-associated infectious risk: a study in a district hospital in Burkina Faso. *25*(2), 219-226.

ISPITS. (2013). Decree No. 2-13-658 on the Instituts Supérieurs des Professions Infirmières et Techniques de Santé (ISPITS).

Kra, O., Aoussi, E., Ehui, I., Ouattara, B., & Bissagnéné, E. J. M. e. M. I. (2009). S-10 Attitudes, knowledge and practices of student nurses regarding nosocomial infections in Abidjan (Côte d'ivoire). *39*, S77-S78.

Liu, L.-M., Curtis, J., & Crookes, P. A. J. J. o. H. I. (2014). Identifying essential infection control competencies for newly graduated nurses: a three-phase study in Australia and Taiwan. *86*(2), 100-109.

Loczenski, B. J. P. Z. (2005). [Hygiene in nursing-1: Hands can transmit invisible dangers]. *58*(7), 432-434.

World Health Organization, O. (2017). Clean care is safer care-The five prongs of the first Global Patient Safety Challenge. In.

Murthy, S. B., Moradiya, Y., Shah, J., Merkler, A. E., Mangat, H. S., Iadacola, C., . . Ziai, W. C. J. N. c. (2016). Nosocomial infections and outcomes after intracerebral hemorrhage: a population-based study. *25*(2), 178-184.

Ndu, A. C., & Arinze-Onyia, S. U. J. M. M. J. (2017). Standard precaution knowledge and adherence: Do Doctors differ from Medical Laboratory Scientists? , *29*(4), 294-300.

Ofili, A., Asuzu, M., & Okojie, O. J. T. N. p. m. j. (2003). Knowledge and practice of universal precautions among nurses in central hospital, Benin-City, Edo State, Nigeria. *10*(1), 26-31.

Ogoina, D., Pondei, K., Adetunji, B., Chima, G., Isichei, C., & Gidado, S. J. J. o. i. p. (2015). Knowledge, attitude and practice of standard precautions of infection control by hospital workers in two tertiary hospitals in Nigeria. *16*(1), 16-22.

Ojulong, J., Mitonga, K. H., & Iipinge, S. J. A. h. s. (2013). Knowledge and attitudes of infection prevention and control among health sciences students at University of Namibia. *13*(4), 1071-1078.

organization, W. H. (2002). Prevention of hospital-acquired infections online Retrieved on October 1, 2009. In.

Organization, W. H. (2005). *WHO recommendations for hand hygiene in health care (advanced version): summary: clean hands are safe hands*. Retrieved from

Pozzetto, B. (2004). MICROORGANISMS RESPONSIBLE FOR NOSOCOMIAL INFECTIONS

Rahiman, F., Chikte, U., & Hughes, G. D. J. N. e. t. (2018). Nursing students' knowledge, attitude and practices of infection prevention and control guidelines at a tertiary institution in the Western Cape: A cross sectional study. *69*, 20-25.

Razine, R., Jroundi, I., Kasouati, J., El Mrabet, M., Sbai, K., Bouaiti, E., . . Benbrahim, N. F. J. R. d. É. e. d. S. P. (2009). Knowledge, attitudes and hand hygiene practices of fifth-year medical students at the CHU Ibn Sina in Rabat, Morocco. *57*, S51.

Samuel, S., Kayode, O., Musa, O., Nwigwe, G., Aboderin, A., Salami, T., . . . microbiology, e. (2010). Nosocomial infections and the challenges of control in developing countries. *11*(2).

SF2H. (2017). the French Society of Hospital Hygiene. (SF2H): Update on Standard Precautions. *66*.

Thakker, V. S., Jadhav, P. R. J. J. o. f. m., & care, p. (2015). Knowledge of hand hygiene in undergraduate medical, dental, and nursing students: A cross-sectional survey. *4*(4), 582.

Trop, M. J. M. T. (2008). Perception du risque nosocomial parmi le personnel hospitalier de l'Hôpital Principal de Dakar. *68*(6), 593-596.

Ward, D. J. J. N. E. T. (2011). The role of education in the prevention and control of infection: a review of the literature. *31*(1), 9-17.

WHO, W. H. O. (2009). WHO Guidelines on Hand Hygiene in Health Care. *52*, 3.

Appendices

Appendix 1: Knowledge score

Questions	Score awarded
General knowledge of nosocomial infections	
What is a nosocomial infection?	1
What factors increase the risk of developing a nosocomial infection?	1
How is nosocomial infection transmitted?	1
Who is the receptive host for nosocomial infections?	1
What is the likely reservoir of nosocomial infection?	1
What microbial agents are involved in hospital-acquired infections?	1
In our Moroccan context, what is the most common nosocomial infection in Morocco?	1
Which body is responsible for preventing nosocomial infections in hospitals, according to the internal regulations of Moroccan hospitals?	3
Total (1)	**10**
Knowledge of attitudes and practices regarding nosocomial infections	
Standard precautions to protect against nosocomial infections are applied with the aim of	2
Standard precautions to protect against nosocomial infections include :	2
Hand hygiene includes	1
Indications for hand hygiene :	1
For you, the benefits of hand washing are :	1
The different types of hand washing are :	1
The purpose of antiseptic washing is to :	1
What is the recommended method for drying hands after washing in the department?	1
The use of gloves should be?	1
We recommend that you keep your gloves on between treatments.	1
Do you need to wash your hands before putting on gloves?	1
What are the indications for using an alcohol-based hand disinfectant (on unsoiled hands)?	1
What is the recommended time for applying hygienic hand rub?	1
Where there is a risk of splashes or sprays of blood and body fluids, care staff must wear ?	1
Is it compulsory to perform perineal cleansing before inserting a urinary catheter?	1
When a bladder catheter is inserted, it is advisable to wear :	1
The nurse's gown must be :	1
How long does the average blouse last?	1
Total (2)	**20**
Total score	**30**

1: General knowledge of nosocomial infections

2: Knowledge of attitudes and practices to prevent nosocomial infection

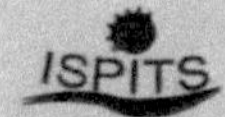

المعهد العالي للمهن التمريضية وتقنيات الصحة، اكادير
Institut Supérieur des Professions Infirmières et Techniques de Santé, Agadir

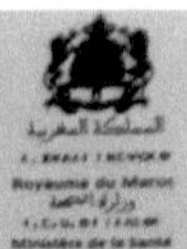

المملكة المغربية
Royaume du Maroc
وزارة الصحة
Ministère de la Santé

A

Monsieur Mohamed Amine BABA

Etudiant inscrit au cycle Master, Filière « Pédagogie des Sciences Infirmières et Techniques de Santé »

Objet : Autorisation pour réaliser une recherche sous le thème « Connaissances, attitudes et pratiques des étudiants en soins infirmiers face aux infections nosocomiales».

Suite à votre demande, nous avons l'honneur de vous informer que la Direction de l'ISPITS d'Agadir vous autorise à réaliser votre étude identifiée ci-dessus, au niveau de l'établissement.

De ce fait, vous êtes appelés, lors de sa réalisation, à respecter scrupuleusement le règlement intérieur de l'institut et les règles d'éthique de la recherche.

De même, vous êtes priés de collaborer et de coordonner avec le responsable de l'Unité de la Gestion Pédagogique/Direction chargée des études, en vue de vous faciliter l'étape de collecte des données auprès de la population estudiantine.

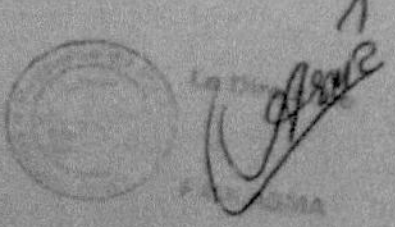

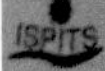

39

Appendix 3: Consent

INFORMATION AND CONSENT FORM

IDENTIFICATION :

Project title :	**Nursing students' knowledge, attitudes and practices regarding nosocomial infections** The case of students at the Institut Supérieur des Professions Infirmières et Techniques de Santé in Agadir

Student-researcher responsible for the project :	
	BABA Mohamed Amine Master's student in nursing and health technology - ISPITSA
Email address :	Babamedamine2@gmail.com

GENERAL AIM OF THE PROJECT AND DIRECTION :

You are invited to take part in this project, the aim of which is to study the level of knowledge of students in the care sector in the face of nosocomial infections, at the ISPITS in AGADIR. This project is being carried out as part of the end-of-study dissertation for the master's degree in nursing education and health techniques, under the supervision of :

- Supervisor: Pr Mohamed NEJMEDDINE, Professor, Agadir Faculty of Science.

- Co-supervisor : Mr Ahmed KHARBACH, Permanent teacher at ISPITS D'AGADIR

    Doctoral student at the Faculty of Medicine and Pharmacy, Rabat.

PROCEDURE(S) OR TASKS REQUIRED OF THE PARTICIPANT :

If you agree to take part in this study, a knowledge assessment questionnaire will be administered. The questionnaire will take approximately 5 to 10 minutes to complete.

ANONYMITY AND CONFIDENTIALITY :

All the information collected in this questionnaire will be treated anonymously and will remain confidential. The results obtained from the processing of this questionnaire may be the subject of scientific publications, but the identity of the participants will not be revealed, nor will any information that could reveal your identity.

THANKS :

Your collaboration is important to the success of this project and we would like to thank you for it.

CONSENT TO PARTICIPATE :

I have read and understood the above information and willingly agree to take part in this research.

Date :	Full name	Signature

<u>**Appendix 4: Questionnaire**</u>

Knowledge of nosocomial infections among students at the Institut Supérieur des Professions Infirmières et Techniques de Santé (Higher Institute for Nursing and Technical Health Professions)

- The case of the nursing care sector

- The results of this survey will be processed anonymously.

- The information collected will be used solely for research purposes.

- Your participation is entirely voluntary and you are guaranteed the right to withdraw.

Student identification

Gender	Feminine ☐ Male ☐
Age	/________/
Option	IP ☐ ISUSI ☐ IAR☐ ISM ☐ ISFSC ☐
Semester :	S4 ☐ S6 ☐
Nationality	Moroccan woman ☐ Foreign ☐
Have you received training in nosocomial infections?	YES ☐ NO ☐
If so, in what academic context?	Basic training ☐ Other context [6]☐

---

[6] Conferences, congresses, workshops ......

What is a nosocomial infection?	☐ Hospital-acquired infection regardless of length of hospital stay ☐ Infection acquired in hospital after 48 h of hospitalisation ☐ Infection acquired in hospital after 24 h of hospitalisation ☐ I don't know
What factors increase the risk of hospital-acquired infection?	☐ Advanced age ☐ Long hospital stay ☐ Prematurity [7]☐ Immunocompromised ☐ I don't know
How is nosocomial infection transmitted?	☐ Handling ☐ Breathing ☐ Cutaneous route ☐ Soiled equipment ☐ Nosocomial infection is not transmissible ☐ I don't know
Who is the receptive host for nosocomial infections?	☐ Neat ☐ Caregiver ☐ Visitors ☐ Carer and cared for ☐ Caregiver and visitors ☐ I don't know
What is the likely reservoir of nosocomial infection?	☐ Caregiver ☐ Caretaker ☐Visitors ☐ Environment ☐ Carer and cared for ☐ Carer, cared for and visitor ☐ Carer, cared for, visitor and environment ☐ I don't know
What microbial agents are involved in hospital-acquired infections?	☐ Bacteria ☐ Virus ☐ Parasite ☐ Fungus ☐ I don't know
In our Moroccan context, what is the most common nosocomial infection in Morocco?	☐Surgical wound infection ☐ Respiratory infection ☐Urinary tract infection ☐ Don't know
Which body is responsible for preventing nosocomial infections in hospitals, according to the internal regulations of Moroccan hospitals?	....

General knowledge of nosocomial infections

---

[7] A newborn weighing less than 1 kg.

Knowledge of attitudes and practices regarding nosocomial infections	
Standard precautions to protect against nosocomial infections are applied with the aim of :	☐ Protect all patients only. ☐ Protect all healthcare staff only. ☐ Protecting all patients and healthcare staff. ☐ I don't know
Standard precautions to protect against nosocomial infections include :	☐ Hand hygiene ☐ Respiratory hygiene ☐ Excreta management ☐ Environmental management ☐ Use of personal protective equipment ☐ AES prevention[8] or any biological product ☐ I don't know
Hand hygiene includes :	☐ Hand washing ☐ Hand disinfection ☐ Both at the same time ☐ I don't know
Indications for hand hygiene :	☐ Before contact with a patient ☐ Before an aseptic procedure [9] ☐ After the risk of exposure to a biological liquid ☐ After contact with a patient ☐ after contact with the patient's environment ☐ I don't know
For you, the benefits of hand washing are :	☐ For self-protection ☐ To protect the patient ☐ Both at the same time ☐ I don't know
The different types of hand washing are :	☐ Simple ☐ antiseptic ☐ surgical ☐ don't know
The purpose of antiseptic washing is to :	☐ Remove only transient germs. ☐ Remove only resident germs.

---

[8] Blood exposure accident
[9] (For example, the insertion of devices such as catheters)

	☐ Suppress transient germs and reduce resident germs. ☐ Don't know
What is the recommended method for drying hands after washing in the department?	☐ Collective towel ☐ Single-use towel ☐ Automatic drying instrument ☐ Don't know
The use of gloves should be?	☐ For each procedure. ☐ Where there is a risk of contact with blood or body fluids /. ☐ Where there is a risk of cutting. ☐ When healthcare workers have a skin lesion.
We recommend that you keep your gloves on between treatments.	Yes ☐ No ☐
Do you need to wash your hands before putting on gloves?	Yes ☐ No ☐
What are the indications for using an alcohol-based hand disinfectant (on unsoiled hands)?	☐ Instead of traditional hand washing ☐ Instead of antiseptic hand washing ☐ Instead of surgical hand washing ☐ Don't know
What is the recommended time for applying hygienic hand rub?	☐ 10 seconds ☐ 15 seconds ☐ 30 seconds ☐ 85 seconds ☐ I don't know
Where there is a risk of splashes or sprays of blood and body fluids, care staff must wear ?	☐ A mask only. ☐ Eye protection only. ☐ Wear a helmet only. ☐ Wear a mask, goggles and a hard hat.
Is it compulsory to perform perineal cleansing before inserting a urinary catheter?	Yes ☐ No ☐
When a bladder catheter is inserted, it is advisable to wear :	Sterile gloves ☐ non-sterile gloves ☐
The nurse's gown must be :	☐ With long sleeves ☐ With short sleeves

How long does the average blouse last?	☐ 1 day ☐ 3 days ☐ 1 week ☐ 2 weeks ☐ 3 weeks ☐ Don't know

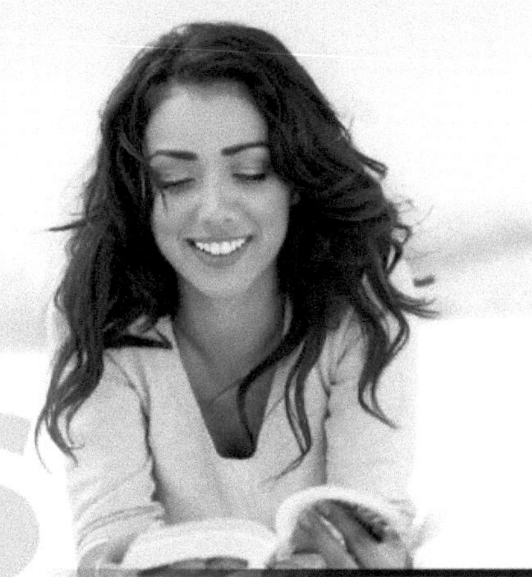

Buy your books fast and straightforward online - at one of world's fastest growing online book stores! Environmentally sound due to Print-on-Demand technologies.

Buy your books online at
www.morebooks.shop

Kaufen Sie Ihre Bücher schnell und unkompliziert online – auf einer der am schnellsten wachsenden Buchhandelsplattformen weltweit! Dank Print-On-Demand umwelt- und ressourcenschonend produziert.

Bücher schneller online kaufen
www.morebooks.shop

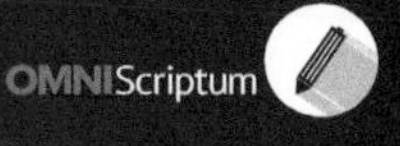

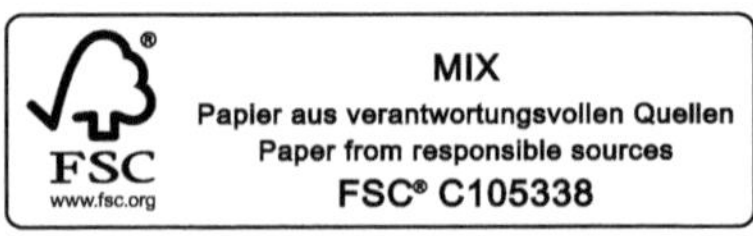

MIX
Papier aus verantwortungsvollen Quellen
Paper from responsible sources
FSC® C105338
FSC
www.fsc.org

Printed by Books on Demand GmbH, Norderstedt / Germany